Contents

Preface

Hello and welcome! If you're in need of guidance on healthy eating, managing your ideal weight, and adopting an active lifestyle, you're in the right place. Before writing this book for you, I delved into years of in-depth research in the fields of nutrition, exercise, and diet. Through discussions with expert dietitians, collaborations with accomplished athletes, listening to the nutritional stories of countless individuals, and embarking on a journey filled with personal experiences, I've decided to share the knowledge and experiences I've gained with you in this book.

The content of our book covers a multitude of important topics that will undoubtedly add value to your life. I've taken care to present these subjects in a clear and comprehensible manner, listing them in bullet points for easy understanding. Understanding and implementing the key aspects of a healthy lifestyle should be accessible to everyone.

It's worth noting that this book is not just for those seeking weight loss. It contains valuable information for anyone who values their health. Whether you're aiming to shed pounds, maintain your current weight, or embrace an energetic and healthy lifestyle, this book will guide you.

Now is the perfect time to start feeling better and reclaiming your health. Let's embark on this journey to a healthier life together, armed with the tips and information we'll be sharing in this book!

What is Healthy Eating?

Healthy eating refers to nourishing your body adequately and in a balanced manner to meet its needs. Healthy eating helps establish and maintain a healthy body weight, reduces the risk of chronic diseases, improves overall health, and contributes to feeling more energetic, vibrant, and content. It's important to note that healthy eating can vary based on factors such as daily energy expenditure, emotional state, stress levels, and body composition.

Healthy eating involves consuming a variety of foods in appropriate quantities and at specific times. A well-balanced diet ensures sufficient intake of essential nutrients such as proteins, carbohydrates, fats, fibers, vitamins, and minerals. Furthermore, consuming foods from natural sources is recommended.

A healthy eating plan involves limiting the consumption of harmful substances like refined sugar, saturated fats, salt, and processed foods. Instead, opting for natural foods such as whole grains, vegetables, fruits, healthy fats, and dairy products is advised.

Healthy eating is important at every age, and it plays a vital role in the healthy growth of children and the graceful aging of adults. A well-designed healthy eating plan forms the foundation of a healthy lifestyle and can assist you in achieving optimal well-being.

Remember, the concept of healthy eating is not rigid; it evolves with individual needs, preferences, and unique circumstances. By making mindful choices and embracing a balanced approach to eating, you can embark on a journey to nourish your body and enhance your overall quality of life.

In our modern society, where fast food and convenience meals are prevalent, it's crucial to take a proactive approach to healthy eating. Educating yourself about the nutritional content of foods, reading labels, and making informed choices can empower you to make positive changes in your diet. Furthermore, understanding portion sizes and practicing mindful eating can help prevent overeating and promote better digestion.

Ultimately, healthy eating is not just a short-term endeavor; it's a lifelong commitment to taking care of your body and prioritizing your well-being. As you navigate the complexities of modern food choices, remember that small, consistent steps can lead to significant improvements in your overall health. By embracing the principles of healthy eating and tailoring them to your individual needs, you're investing in a healthier and happier future.

The Significance of Food Groups in Achieving a Balanced and Healthy Diet

A balanced and healthy diet is a cornerstone of overall well-being, and understanding the role of different food groups is key to achieving this nutritional harmony. Food groups provide essential nutrients that fuel our bodies, support growth, and maintain optimal health. Let's delve deeper into the importance of each food group and how they collectively contribute to a well-rounded diet.

Proteins: Proteins are the building blocks of life, playing a pivotal role in tissue repair, immune function, and enzyme production. They consist of amino acids, which are essential for numerous bodily processes. Animal sources like lean meats, poultry, fish, and dairy products provide complete proteins containing all essential amino acids. Plant-based sources such as legumes, beans, nuts, and seeds offer valuable protein options as well. Incorporating a variety of protein sources ensures a comprehensive intake of amino acids that are vital for muscle maintenance, immune strength, and cellular repair.

Carbohydrates: Carbohydrates are the primary energy source for our bodies, supplying glucose that powers cellular functions and fuels physical activities. They can be categorized into simple carbohydrates found in fruits, sugars, and refined grains, as well as complex carbohydrates present in whole grains, vegetables, and legumes. Whole grains, such as brown rice, quinoa, and whole wheat bread, provide sustained energy due to their higher fiber content, promoting better blood sugar control and digestive health.

Fats: Dietary fats are essential for energy storage, insulation, and protection of vital organs. While fats have long been associated with negative connotations, it's important to differentiate between healthy fats and trans fats or saturated fats. Unsaturated fats found in avocados, nuts, seeds, and olive oil are heart-healthy options that support cholesterol regulation and overall cardiovascular health. Moderation is key, as fats are calorie-dense and excessive intake can lead to weight gain.

Fiber: Fiber is the unsung hero of digestion, aiding in regular bowel movements and preventing constipation. Both soluble and insoluble fiber contribute to gut health, promote satiety, and assist in maintaining a healthy weight.

Whole grains, fruits, vegetables, legumes, and nuts are excellent sources of fiber, and incorporating them into your diet can have a positive impact on digestive wellness and overall vitality.

Vitamins and Minerals: Vitamins and minerals act as catalysts for various biochemical reactions in the body, supporting everything from bone health and immune function to wound healing and energy production. Each vitamin and mineral has a specific role, and a diverse diet rich in fruits, vegetables, whole grains, lean proteins, and dairy products ensures you receive the necessary spectrum of these micronutrients.

In summary, a truly balanced and healthy diet involves embracing the synergistic contributions of all food groups. A diverse and colorful plate, filled with lean proteins, whole grains, healthy fats, and a plethora of fruits and vegetables, ensures that you receive a wide range of nutrients. It's essential to tailor your nutritional choices to your individual needs, keeping in mind factors such as age, activity level, and any specific health conditions. By appreciating the value of each food group and making conscious choices, you pave the way for a vibrant and nourished life.

Calculating Calories and Macro-Nutrient Distribution: A Comprehensive Approach to a Balanced Diet

Embarking on a journey toward a balanced and healthy diet involves a multifaceted understanding of caloric intake and the distribution of macro-nutrients. These fundamental aspects are the cornerstones of crafting an eating plan that supports your overall well-being and specific goals.

Understanding Calories: Calories serve as the measure of energy contained in the foods we consume. This energy is essential for fueling bodily functions, maintaining cellular activities, and enabling physical activities. The total number of calories we consume directly affects our body weight—consuming more calories than we expend leads to weight gain, while a calorie deficit results in weight loss. Calculating your daily caloric needs is influenced by several factors, including basal metabolic rate (BMR), physical activity level, age, gender, and overall health. It's essential to strike a balance between calorie intake and expenditure to achieve your desired health outcomes.

Macro-Nutrient Distribution: Equally significant is the distribution of macro-nutrients within your daily caloric intake. Macro-nutrients—protein, carbohydrates, and fats—serve distinct functions and are vital for various bodily processes.

Protein: Often regarded as the body's building blocks, proteins are indispensable for tissue repair, muscle maintenance, and immune function. Protein intake is crucial for both active individuals aiming to build muscle and those seeking to maintain their overall health.

Aiming for 10-35% of your daily caloric intake from protein sources like lean meats, poultry, fish, dairy products, legumes, and plant-based options such as tofu and tempeh ensures that your body receives the essential amino acids required for optimal functioning.

Carbohydrates: Carbohydrates are the primary energy source for your body, playing a central role in fueling daily activities and workouts. They can be classified as simple carbohydrates found in sugars and refined products and complex carbohydrates found in whole grains, vegetables, and fruits. Striking a balance between both forms is essential for maintaining steady blood sugar levels and sustaining energy throughout the day. Carbohydrates should generally contribute 45-65% of your daily caloric intake, depending on your activity level and goals.

Fats: Fats are often misunderstood but are vital for various functions, including hormone production, insulation, and the absorption of fat-soluble vitamins. Opting for healthy fats, such as those found in avocados, nuts, seeds, and fatty fish like salmon, supports cardiovascular health and overall well-being. Healthy fats should constitute around 20-35% of your daily caloric intake, with saturated fats limited to prevent negative health implications.

Creating an optimal macro-nutrient distribution depends on individual factors such as age, gender, body composition, and activity level. Tailoring your nutritional intake to meet your specific needs ensures that your body operates efficiently and effectively. However, it's important to note that rigidly adhering to a specific macro ratio may not suit everyone; flexibility and adjustment based on progress and personal goals are key.

In summary, a balanced diet encompasses the careful management of calories and macro-nutrient distribution. Achieving this balance requires a holistic understanding of your body's unique requirements, activity level, and objectives. Consulting with a qualified dietitian or nutritionist can provide valuable insights tailored to your individual needs, helping you pave the way for long-term health, vitality, and success.

Mastering the Art of Diet Planning and Cultivating Nourishing Eating Habits

The journey to a healthier you begins with meticulous diet planning and the cultivation of mindful eating habits. These twin pillars lay the foundation for achieving your wellness aspirations, empowering you to take charge of your nutrition and overall health.

Strategizing Your Diet Plan: The essence of a successful diet plan lies in meticulous strategizing.

Begin by assessing your individual goals—whether it's weight management, muscle gain, or overall well-being. Once you have a clear objective in mind, calculate your daily caloric needs considering factors like basal metabolic rate (BMR), physical activity level, and goals. Design your meals to align with these caloric requirements while ensuring a balanced distribution of macro-nutrients. While trends like intermittent fasting have gained popularity for their potential benefits, it's essential to personalize your approach based on your body's response and your specific goals.

Inquisitive Label Reading: An invaluable skill in your nutritional toolkit is the ability to decipher food labels. Delve beyond the alluring packaging to understand the nutritional breakdown of the food you're consuming. Pay attention to portion sizes and servings, as these often impact the calorie content significantly. Keeping track of your daily intake not only facilitates accurate caloric tracking but also provides insights into the macro-nutrient composition of your diet.

Navigating Towards Nutrient-Rich Choices: The heart of a healthy diet plan is the deliberate selection of nutrient-rich foods. Embrace the spectrum of colorful fruits and vegetables, lean proteins, whole grains, and healthy fats. These foods are dense in vitamins, minerals, and phytochemicals, nourishing your body at the cellular level. Remember that nutrient-rich doesn't equate to flavorless—experiment with herbs, spices, and healthy cooking techniques to create delectable and healthful meals.

Evolving Portion Control: Portion control is a powerful tool that empowers you to savor your favorite foods while maintaining calorie balance. Opt for mindful portion sizes by using smaller plates, allowing you to visually appreciate a full plate even with smaller portions. Eating slowly encourages heightened satiety and provides your brain ample time to signal fullness, potentially preventing overindulgence.

The Hydration Game: Hydration is a fundamental aspect of health, often overlooked in the realm of dietary planning. Water is the elixir of life, supporting digestion, nutrient absorption, and overall bodily functions. Prioritize water consumption, and consider infusing it with fruits or herbs to enhance its appeal. Be cautious with sugary beverages and caffeinated drinks, as they can contribute to unnecessary calories and hinder optimal hydration.

Progressive Goal Setting:

Successful diet planning thrives on achievable and measurable goals. Set objectives that are specific, measurable, attainable, relevant, and time-bound (SMART). Break down your journey into short-term and long-term targets, celebrating each milestone achieved. This approach not only enhances motivation but also fosters a sense of accomplishment.

Mindful Eating Rituals:

Cultivating mindful eating habits transforms your relationship with food. Engage all your senses during meals, appreciating the colors, textures, and flavors. Eating in a calm environment, free from distractions, allows you to connect with your body's hunger and fullness cues. Chew each bite deliberately, promoting optimal digestion and satisfaction.

Holistic Harmony: Diet planning and adopting nourishing eating habits are interwoven elements of a holistic approach to health. Consider complementing your efforts with regular physical activity, be it a brisk walk, yoga, or strength training. Engaging in activities you enjoy fosters a sustainable and positive relationship with exercise. Additionally, managing stress through relaxation techniques, meditation, or hobbies can significantly impact your digestive health and overall well-being.

In essence, the art of diet planning and cultivating wholesome eating habits is a journey of self-discovery and empowerment. It's about embracing nutrition as a tool to fuel your aspirations, promote vitality, and celebrate the wonder of a well-nourished body and mind.

The Dynamic Trio: Navigating Protein, Carbohydrates, and Fats in Your Dietary Odyssey

Embarking on a journey towards a healthier you involves navigating the intricate landscape of nutrition, where the triumvirate of protein, carbohydrates, and fats takes center stage. These three macronutrients are the pillars upon which your body's vitality, function, and resilience are built. Let's delve into the multifaceted realm of each nutrient:

1. Protein Proficiency: Protein, often hailed as the body's architectural marvel, serves as the bedrock for growth, repair, and sustenance. It plays a pivotal role in maintaining lean muscle mass, strengthening bones, bolstering the immune system, and facilitating enzymatic reactions. Moreover, protein has a unique satiating effect, taming hunger pangs and promoting a feeling of fullness. The tapestry of protein sources is vast and includes lean meats, poultry, fish, dairy products, eggs, legumes, nuts, seeds, and the versatile soy products. The art of integrating protein effectively lies in both variety and balance.

2. Carbohydrate Chronicles:

Carbohydrates, often dubbed the body's primary energy source, are a cornerstone of daily vitality. They can be likened to the fuel that propels your physical endeavors. However, the quality of carbohydrates is a critical determinant of their impact. Wholesome sources such as whole grains, colorful vegetables, and fiber-rich fruits provide a steady release of energy while nurturing digestive health. It's imperative to steer clear of the abyss of refined sugars and processed carbohydrates, which can lead to spikes in blood sugar, weight gain, and metabolic imbalances.

3. Fats: The Unsung Heroes:

Fats, a category long plagued by misconceptions, are integral to optimal bodily function. They're not only a potent energy reserve but also act as guardians for vital organs and facilitate the absorption of fat-soluble vitamins. Embracing the nuances of fats involves differentiating between the champions and the adversaries. Healthy fats, prevalent in avocados, olive oil, fatty fish, nuts, and seeds, have been shown to support cardiovascular health, brain function, and inflammation management. On the flip side, trans fats and excessive saturated fats are the antagonists, potentially culminating in cardiovascular woes and metabolic derailments.

Within the mosaic of macronutrients, crafting a nourishing diet plan transcends merely understanding their roles—it involves their harmonious integration into your daily regimen. Synchronizing their intake in alignment with your individual needs and goals paves the way for a holistic approach to well-being.

Furthermore, the concept of portion control is an art form within itself. It entails appreciating the balance between satisfying your body's requirements and avoiding excess. Portion sizes, often influenced by cultural norms and visual cues, require a mindful approach to prevent overconsumption while honoring your hunger.

Remember, the tapestry of protein, carbohydrates, and fats is interwoven with the threads of moderation, variety, and quality. Consulting a registered dietitian or nutrition expert can provide you with personalized insights into optimizing this dynamic interplay. As you navigate the intricacies of nutrition, let the synergy of these three macronutrients be the compass guiding you towards an energized, vibrant, and balanced life.

Navigating the Supplement Galaxy: A Deeper Dive into Vitamins and Minerals

As we traverse the realm of nutrition, the spotlight shines on the captivating universe of vitamins and minerals—essential components that orchestrate the symphony of bodily functions. While a balanced diet aims to deliver these micronutrients, there are instances when vitamin and mineral supplements can be instrumental in fortifying our nutritional armor.

1. The Sunlit Vitamin D: Vitamin D, often referred to as the "sunshine vitamin," is a multifaceted nutrient that plays a pivotal role in bone health, immune function, and more. Synthesized when your skin interacts with sunlight, its production can wane in the shadows of limited sunlight exposure. Individuals in regions with extended winters or those with indoor lifestyles may benefit from supplementation. It's a testament to the intricate interplay between nature and science—an ode to our innate connection with the cosmos.

2. Iron: The Essential Cog: Iron, an elemental force within our physiology, is an essential component of hemoglobin—a protein that carries oxygen from the lungs to tissues throughout the body. Those prone to iron deficiency—anemia—such as menstruating women, pregnant individuals, and children, may find their nutritional landscape enhanced by iron supplements. The challenge lies in striking a delicate balance; an excess can be as detrimental as a deficiency.

3. The Omega-3 Odyssey:

Embarking on a voyage to cardiovascular well-being unveils the importance of omega-3 fatty acids. These remarkable compounds, found abundantly in fatty fish, walnuts, and flaxseeds, exhibit anti-inflammatory properties and contribute to heart health. The maritime narrative extends to supplements, allowing individuals to navigate these nutritional waters regardless of dietary preferences.

Yet, the art of embracing supplements demands discernment and respect for moderation. It's akin to crafting a personalized constellation—an intricate blend of dietary sources and supplemental support. The symphony of micronutrients can achieve harmonious resonance when fueled by knowledge and guided by experts.

In the pursuit of enhanced well-being, understanding the symbiotic dance between your dietary choices and supplemental endeavors is paramount. A collaboration with a qualified dietitian or healthcare professional illuminates the path, ensuring that your supplement selections align with your unique nutritional needs.

A word of wisdom—a robust dietary foundation enriched with whole foods, encompassing a rainbow of colors and nutrients, forms the bedrock of a thriving existence. The supplements, like celestial companions, offer an extra dimension—a cosmic interplay between science and nature—to fortify the vibrant tapestry of your health journey.

The Art of Harnessing Diets: Utilization, Wisdom, and Beyond

The world of diets is a complex landscape, offering a spectrum of possibilities for achieving health, vitality, and specific wellness goals. Yet, amidst this vast expanse, the key to unlocking the true potential of diets lies in their proper utilization and the wisdom to discern what resonates with your unique journey. Here, we delve deeper into the nuanced facets of diet utilization and the profound wisdom that accompanies it.

1. Elevate Awareness and Mindful Eating: A cornerstone of effective diet utilization is cultivating mindfulness around your eating habits. Mindful eating involves savoring each bite, tuning into your body's hunger and fullness cues, and appreciating the textures and flavors of your meals. This practice not only enhances your connection with food but also aids in portion control and prevents overindulgence.

2. Embrace Nutrient-Rich Diversity: Within the realm of diets, the tapestry of nutrient-rich foods paints a vivid canvas of possibilities. A vibrant array of fruits, vegetables, whole grains, lean proteins, and healthy fats provides your body with an orchestra of vitamins, minerals, antioxidants, and phytochemicals. This diversity is your passport to optimal health, bolstering your immune system, enhancing your energy levels, and fortifying your overall well-being.

3. Navigate the Myth of "Good" vs. "Bad" Foods: The dichotomy of "good" and "bad" foods oversimplifies the intricate relationship we have with nutrition. Instead of labeling foods, focus on the overall quality of your diet. Balancing occasional indulgences with predominantly nutrient-dense choices enables you to relish life's culinary pleasures while honoring your health.

4. Empower with Education: An empowered journey through diets is paved with knowledge. Understanding how different nutrients function in your body, deciphering food labels, and distinguishing between credible nutritional information and fads equip you with the tools to make informed choices. The empowerment that comes from education ensures that your dietary decisions align with your goals.

5. Holistic Wellness Beyond the Plate: A holistic approach to dieting extends beyond the realm of food. Adequate sleep, stress management, and positive social connections are essential threads in the tapestry of well-being. A sound mind and soul harmonize with a nourished body to create a symphony of vitality.

6. Seek Professional Guidance: Navigating the labyrinth of diets can be complex, and seeking the guidance of a registered dietitian or nutrition expert can provide invaluable insights. These professionals consider your individual needs, preferences, and health conditions, crafting a personalized roadmap that propels you toward your wellness aspirations.

In this grand symphony of diet utilization and wisdom, remember that your journey is as unique as your fingerprints. The key lies in embracing an approach that resonates with your values, prioritizing self-compassion over perfection, and honoring the intricate dance between your body, mind, and spirit. The path to harnessing diets becomes a voyage of self-discovery, empowerment, and a celebration of your quest for lasting health and vitality.

A Comprehensive Approach to Effective Weight Management and Balance

In the pursuit of weight loss and maintaining a healthy weight, it's essential to adopt a holistic approach that considers various factors beyond just calorie counting and exercise. Achieving sustainable results involves a multi-faceted strategy that encompasses dietary choices, physical activity, mental well-being, and long-term commitment.

1. Caloric Balance and Deficit:
The cornerstone of successful weight management revolves around understanding caloric balance. Creating a caloric deficit—where your body expends more calories than it consumes—initiates weight loss. However, the focus should be on a moderate deficit that allows for gradual, sustainable changes, as extreme calorie restriction can have adverse effects on metabolism and overall health.

2. Embrace Dietary Diversity:
Rather than adhering to restrictive diets, prioritizing dietary diversity is key. A well-rounded intake of macronutrients, including protein, carbohydrates, and healthy fats,

ensures your body receives essential nutrients for optimal functioning. Incorporating a variety of fruits, vegetables, whole grains, lean proteins, and plant-based sources fosters satiety and supports overall well-being.

3. Opt for Healthy Fats: Healthy fats play a pivotal role in weight management. Unsaturated fats, found in foods like avocados, nuts, seeds, and olive oil, not only contribute to heart health but also aid in curbing hunger and promoting satisfaction after meals.

4. The Significance of Hydration: Proper hydration is often underestimated in weight management. Water not only quenches your body's thirst but also supports metabolic processes and can help prevent overeating. Choosing water as your primary beverage while reducing the intake of sugary drinks supports weight management efforts.

5. Exercise Regimen: Establishing a consistent exercise routine is instrumental in achieving and maintaining a healthy weight. Incorporating a combination of cardiovascular exercises, such as brisk walking or cycling, and strength training enhances muscle mass, boosts metabolism, and helps with calorie expenditure. Tailoring your exercise plan to your preferences and goals ensures long-term adherence.

6. Psychological Well-Being:

Recognizing the psychological aspects of weight management is crucial. Cultivating a positive mindset and practicing self-compassion are essential components of your journey. Setting realistic expectations, celebrating small victories, and maintaining a healthy relationship with food are pivotal for sustained success.

7. Long-Term Perspective:

Successful weight management is not a short-term endeavor. Prioritizing gradual progress over quick fixes ensures lasting results. Creating achievable short-term goals and focusing on overall well-being rather than solely on the scale fosters a balanced and positive approach.

In essence, effective weight management is not solely about shedding pounds; it's about cultivating a healthy lifestyle that promotes well-being. By embracing a comprehensive strategy that encompasses nutrition, exercise, mental wellness, and sustainable habits, you can achieve your weight management goals while fostering an improved quality of life. Remember, each individual's journey is unique, so customize your approach to suit your preferences, needs, and aspirations.

Synergizing Exercise and Diet for Optimal Health

Achieving optimal health involves a holistic approach that encompasses both exercise and diet. These two components work in tandem to create a strong foundation for well-being. By understanding the intricate relationship between exercise and diet, individuals can unlock a multitude of benefits that extend beyond physical appearance to encompass mental, emotional, and overall health.

1. The Science of Synergy: The interplay between exercise and diet is grounded in science. Engaging in physical activity increases energy expenditure, creating a greater demand for nutrients to support recovery and muscle growth. A well-balanced diet, rich in essential nutrients, provides the raw materials necessary for these processes to occur efficiently. Nutrient-dense foods fuel exercise performance, while exercise enhances the body's ability to absorb and utilize these nutrients.

2. Weight Management: The synergy between exercise and diet plays a pivotal role in weight management. A balanced diet contributes to caloric control and provides the energy needed for workouts. Regular exercise increases the body's metabolic rate, enabling the efficient burning of calories and helping to create a caloric deficit necessary for weight loss. This combination promotes healthy and sustainable weight management.

3. Muscle Development: Exercise stimulates muscle growth, but the process requires adequate protein intake from the diet. Protein is essential for muscle repair and recovery, making it an indispensable component of post-workout nutrition. Engaging in resistance training, such as weightlifting, complements a protein-rich diet, leading to enhanced muscle development and definition.

4. Cardiovascular Health:

Cardiovascular exercises like running, swimming, and cycling challenge the heart and lungs, leading to improved cardiovascular fitness. A balanced diet, notably one low in saturated and trans fats, supports heart health by maintaining healthy cholesterol levels and reducing the risk of cardiovascular diseases. Consuming nutrient-rich foods rich in antioxidants and omega-3 fatty acids also promotes heart health.

5. Mental and Emotional Well-being: The synergy between

exercise and diet extends to mental and emotional well-being. Physical activity triggers the release of endorphins, which contribute to feelings of happiness and reduced stress. A diet rich in vitamins, minerals, and omega-3 fatty acids supports brain health and cognitive function, positively impacting mood and mental clarity.

6. Long-Term Sustainability:

Incorporating exercise and a balanced diet into daily life fosters a sustainable lifestyle. Crash diets and extreme exercise regimens are often short-lived and yield temporary results. In contrast, a consistent and well-rounded approach to both exercise and diet promotes long-term adherence, leading to lasting health benefits.

7. Personalization is Key: Each individual's exercise and dietary needs are unique. Factors such as age, fitness level, goals, and health conditions must be considered when designing a personalized plan. Consulting with professionals such as personal trainers and registered dietitians can help tailor a program that aligns with individual needs.

In conclusion, the integration of exercise and diet forms the cornerstone of a healthy lifestyle. Recognizing the synergistic effects of these two components allows individuals to harness their combined power for improved physical, mental, and emotional well-being. This comprehensive approach sets the stage for lifelong health and vitality, emphasizing that adopting positive habits in both exercise and diet is not a short-term endeavor, but a lifelong commitment to nurturing a healthier and happier self.

The Art of Meal Preparation: A Comprehensive Guide to Nurturing a Healthy Lifestyle

Navigating the realm of healthy eating can sometimes feel like a daunting task, but armed with the right strategies and a dash of culinary creativity, meal preparation can become your secret weapon for achieving your nutritional goals. Beyond the mere act of cooking, meal prep is a holistic approach that empowers you to make intentional and well-informed choices about the foods you consume. Let's delve into the intricacies of meal preparation and explore how you can master the art of crafting nourishing and delightful meals.

1. Methodical Planning and Strategic Preparation: The cornerstone of effective meal preparation is thoughtful planning. Dedicate time to curate a weekly meal plan that aligns with your dietary objectives and lifestyle. Factor in your nutritional requirements, portion sizes, and personal preferences. Create a detailed shopping list based on your plan, ensuring you have all the necessary ingredients on hand. This methodical approach minimizes impulse decisions and sets you up for success throughout the week.

2. The Symphony of Flavors and Textures: Elevate your meals by embracing a diverse array of ingredients. Incorporate a rainbow of colorful vegetables, whole grains, lean proteins, and healthy fats. Experiment with various cooking techniques to enhance flavors and textures. Roasting vegetables brings out their natural sweetness, while grilling imparts a delightful smokiness. These culinary nuances not only tantalize your taste buds but also amplify the nutritional value of your meals.

3. Prepping with Purpose:

Strategic meal preparation involves much more than chopping vegetables and assembling ingredients. It's about setting the stage for efficient cooking. Consider marinating proteins in flavorful concoctions, such as citrus and herbs, to infuse them with delectable tastes. Batch-cook staple foods like quinoa, brown rice, or grilled chicken, which can serve as versatile building blocks for a variety of meals throughout the week.

4. Harnessing the Power of Portions: Portion control is a fundamental aspect of meal prep that supports both weight

management and balanced nutrition. Invest in portion-sized containers to effortlessly divide meals. By controlling portion sizes, you gain a better understanding of your caloric intake and foster mindful eating habits.

5. Cultivating Creativity with Leftovers: Embrace the art of repurposing leftovers to prevent food waste and stimulate culinary creativity. Transform yesterday's roasted vegetables into a nourishing grain bowl, or blend surplus cooked quinoa into a protein-packed breakfast parfait. Embracing leftovers invites innovation into your kitchen and bolsters sustainability efforts.

6. Efficient Cooking Techniques:

Exploring different cooking methods can significantly influence the nutritional profile of your meals. Consider incorporating techniques such as steaming, sautéing, baking, or sous-vide cooking. These methods retain nutrients, preserve natural flavors, and minimize the need for excessive fats or oils.

7. The Empowerment of Preparation: Beyond its nutritional merits, meal preparation empowers you to take ownership of your dietary choices. As you become attuned to the ingredients in your meals, you can make informed decisions that align with your

health and wellness goals. This newfound sense of control instills confidence in your ability to nourish your body optimally.

In essence, meal preparation is a symphony of planning, creativity, and intentionality. It transcends the realm of cooking to become a holistic approach to nurturing your body and mind. By embracing the nuances of meal prep, you embark on a journey of mindful consumption, culinary exploration, and personal empowerment—a journey that promises to enrich your well-being and transform the way you relate to food.

My Success Story: A Journey of Transformation and Willpower

In life, there are moments that mark turning points. If you haven't experienced such a moment yet, I hope my story serves as an inspiration for you to take significant steps toward a healthier lifestyle. My story revolves around a transformation that began in my high school years and celebrates the triumph of willpower. This tale exemplifies that a healthy life is attainable and change is possible for everyone.

The first turning point in my life occurred during my high school years when my physical appearance began to bother me. Despite my height of 180 cm, I weighed only 55 kilograms. This situation manifested as sunken cheeks, darkened under-eye circles, and visible veins. The reactions of my friends to these changes acted as a catalyst for my internal transformation. I started researching healthy eating and exercise. After endless hours of watching videos and reading articles, I came to understand that healthy weight gain requires a balanced diet and consistent exercise. I increased my caloric intake and began experimenting with exercise routines.

My journey commenced with regular home workouts. As I maintained discipline, I discovered that difficulties gradually diminished. Joining a gym further amplified my motivation. Starting my 11th-grade summer vacation at 55 kilograms, I concluded it weighing 75 kilograms. The most gratifying aspect was the positive reactions from my friends. I had embarked on a new phase, successfully molding my life through the power of change.

When I entered university, new challenges arose in maintaining a healthy lifestyle. Managing weight gain became more complex. However, a roommate showed me that even university life can be disciplined. Over two years, intermittent fasting, morning cardio, balanced nutrition, and consistent exercise became part of my routine. This period allowed me to understand my body better and accumulate valuable experiences in these domains.

As university came to an end, my journey was far from over. I dedicated myself more to sports and healthy eating, continuously seeking to expand my knowledge and expertise. Now, I continue to pursue exercise and nutritious eating, always striving for self-improvement. This story underscores the substantial impact of willpower in catalyzing significant change and highlights the consistent effort required for a healthy lifestyle. Change is attainable for everyone, and this narrative stands as proof of that principle.

Conclusion: A Guiding Light Towards a Healthier Life

This book represents the culmination of an extensive effort, where I've compiled and curated the knowledge gained from my research, personal experiences, and observations of others' lives. My intention was to present the information in a clear and comprehensive manner. I've organized the content into succinct points and structured it with informative headings. This work serves as a reservoir of invaluable insights for individuals embarking on their journey towards healthier nutrition and exercise habits.

The content within this book is intended to guide and illuminate the path for those looking to delve into the realms of healthier eating and active living. Every piece of information provided here has been thoughtfully selected to equip you with the tools necessary for making informed decisions about your health and wellness. The importance of cultivating these habits cannot be overstated, and I hope that the guidance presented here helps you navigate this transformative journey.

I extend my heartfelt gratitude to you for investing your time in exploring the pages of this book. Your commitment to learning and bettering yourself is truly commendable. As you embark on your path towards a healthier lifestyle, remember that it's not just about the destination, but also the journey itself. May you find the strength, motivation, and joy in adopting healthier habits, and may these changes lead you to a life filled with vitality and well-being.

Wishing you all the best on your journey to a healthier and happier life.